# 2-WEEKS

# BELLY

# FAT BUSTER

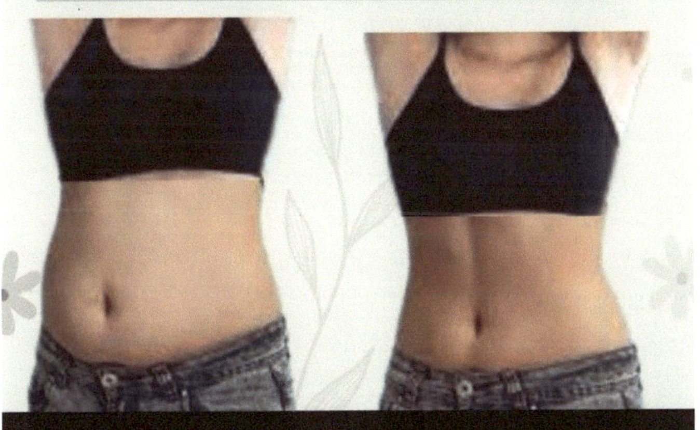

# DEDICATION

To those who struggle with visceral fat accumulation and the health complications that accompany it: This book is dedicated to you. You are not alone in your journey, and you have the power to make positive changes in your life. May this book serve as a guide and a source of inspiration as you strive to improve your health and well-being.

# TABLE OF CONTENTS

# ACKNOWLEDGMENTS

I would like to express my sincere gratitude to everyone who contributed to the creation of this book. First, I would like to thank my family and friends for their support and encouragement throughout this journey. I am also grateful to the healthcare professionals, wellness coaches, and researchers who shared their knowledge and insights on visceral fat accumulation. Finally, I would like to acknowledge the many people who bravely shared their personal stories of struggling with this issue. Your courage and strength have inspired me to share this book with the world.

# CHAPTER ONE

# INTRODUCTION:

## The basics of visceral fat

Did you know that one of the biggest risk factors for chronic diseases like heart disease and diabetes is a condition called visceral fat (obesity)? Visceral obesity is fat that wraps around your abdominal organs deep inside your body, you may not always feel it or see it. In some cases like TOFI you may have a flat tummy and still have visceral fat.

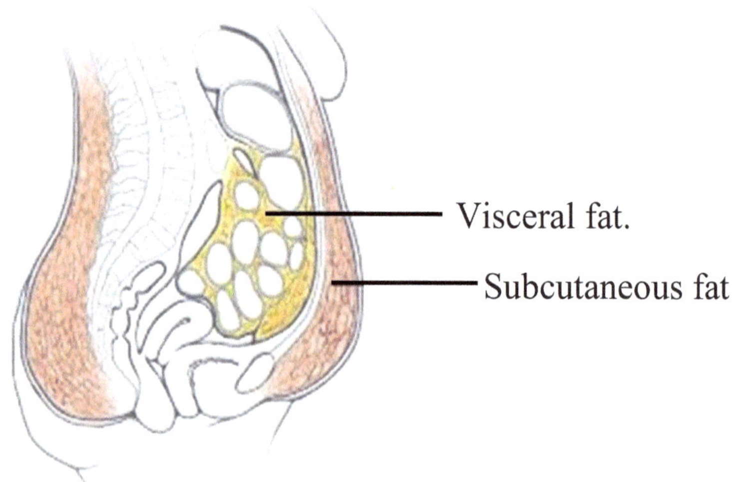

This visceral fat could lead to serious health problems. This book will show you how to reduce visceral fat through diet, exercise, and lifestyle changes. You'll learn about the health risks of visceral fat, and get a step-by-step plan to help you achieve your goals.

## WHY IT'S IMPORTANT TO REDUCE VISCERAL FAT?

Excessive body fat is bad to your health, but when compared to the subcutaneous fat the visceral kind is more likely to raise your risk for serious medical issues. Heart disease, Alzheimer's, type 2 diabetes, stroke, and high cholesterol are some of the conditions that are strongly linked to too much fat in your trunk. Researchers suspect that visceral fat makes more of certain proteins that inflame your body's tissues and organs and narrow your <u>blood</u> vessels. That can make your <u>blood pressure</u> go up and cause other problems.

**HEART DISEASE:** Visceral fat increases the risk of developing coronary artery disease, this is when the arteries that supply blood to the heart become narrowed or blocked. Visceral fat can contribute to atherosclerosis, which is when fatty deposits build up in the arteries. These deposits can cause the arteries to narrow, which can restrict blood flow. This can lead to a number of problems, including heart attack and stroke. Well, as we mentioned, visceral fat can increase the risk of heart attack and stroke by contributing to atherosclerosis. But there are other ways that visceral fat can increase the risk of these conditions as well. For example, visceral fat can cause inflammation, which can damage the heart and blood vessels. Visceral fat can also increase levels of certain hormones that can cause the blood to clot more easily, which can lead to a heart attack or stroke.

**High Blood Pressure:** Visceral fat can cause the body to release more of a hormone called **angiotensin,** which causes the blood vessels to narrow and the blood pressure to rise. This can eventually lead to hypertension, or high blood pressure, which is a major risk factor for heart disease and stroke.

**High Cholesterol** is another condition that's closely

linked to visceral fat. Visceral fat can cause the liver to produce more cholesterol than usual, which can lead to high levels of bad cholesterol in the blood. Bad cholesterol, or LDL cholesterol, can build up in the arteries and contribute to atherosclerosis, which we talked about before. It can also increase the risk of heart attack and stroke.

Visceral fat can lead to **Inflammation:** As we mentioned before, visceral fat can cause the body to release inflammatory substances. These substances can cause inflammation throughout the body, including in the blood vessels, heart, and liver. Inflammation can damage these organs and increase the risk of cardiovascular disease. Are you still with me?

**Type 2 Diabetes:** The link between visceral fat and type 2 diabetes is complex, but we'll try to explain it simply. Visceral fat causes the body to release hormones and inflammatory substances that can damage the insulin-producing cells in the pancreas. This can lead to a condition called insulin resistance, which means that the body doesn't respond properly to the hormone insulin. Insulin resistance can eventually cause the blood sugar levels to rise, leading to type 2 diabetes.

As we said, visceral fat can cause the body to release inflammatory substances. One of these substances is called tumor necrosis factor (TNF). TNF has been linked to insulin resistance and can also cause the liver to produce more glucose, which can lead to high blood sugar levels. TNF can also cause the liver to produce more cholesterol and fatty acids, which can contribute to weight gain and obesity. So, visceral fat is clearly a major risk factor for type 2 diabetes.

**Brain And Mental Health:** Visceral fat can cause inflammation in the brain, leading to cognitive decline and an increased risk of depression. It can also affect the levels of serotonin and dopamine in the brain, which can lead to anxiety and other mental health issues. So, visceral fat not only affects physical health, but it can also have a negative impact on mental health.

# CHAPTER TWO

# HEALTHY EATING HABITS

Many people eat more than they need to, leading to weight gain and an increase in visceral fat. A good rule of thumb is to eat until you're satisfied, not stuffed. Eating slowly and mindfully can also help you pay attention to when you're full. Another important aspect of healthy eating is to focus on eating a variety of nutrient-rich foods. This includes eating plenty of fruits, vegetables, whole grains, and lean proteins. Another aspect of a healthy diet: meal timing. Some research suggests that eating your largest meal earlier in the day, and then having smaller meals or snacks throughout the rest of the day, may help reduce visceral fat. This is called "eating with the circadian rhythm."

# <u>NOTE:</u>

- One strategy is to focus on eating more "mindfully." This means paying attention to your food, savoring each bite, and stopping when you're satisfied. Another strategy is to plan your meals ahead of time. This can help you avoid making unhealthy choices when you're hungry. And finally, remember to drink plenty of water! Water can help you feel full and satisfied. Do you think these strategies are doable?

- Another key strategy is to limit processed foods and added sugars. Processed foods, like frozen meals and packaged snacks, often contain unhealthy amounts of sugar, salt, and fat.

Instead, focus on eating more whole, unprocessed foods. As for added sugars, try to limit them to no more than 10% of your daily calories. This will help you avoid unnecessary calories and reduce your risk of chronic diseases. Do you think you can make these changes to your diet?

- Another key part of a healthy diet is to make sure you're getting enough protein. Protein helps you feel full and satisfied, and it also helps maintain muscle mass. Good sources of protein include fish, poultry, eggs, legumes, and nuts. Try to include some protein at each meal. How does that sound?

## Recipes that can help reduce visceral fat.

1. **Lean beef:** Lean beef is a great source of protein, and it also contains a type of fat called conjugated linoleic acid (CLA). CLA has been shown to reduce visceral fat in some studies. Other good sources of CLA include full-fat dairy products, such as whole milk and cheese.

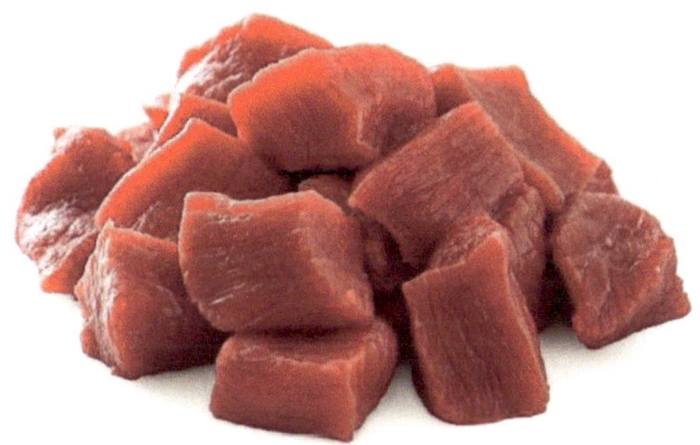

As I mentioned, lean beef is a good source of CLA, which has been shown to reduce visceral fat. CLA works by inhibiting the activity of certain enzymes that cause fat storage. It also increases the breakdown of fat cells. So, incorporating lean beef into your diet can help reduce visceral fat over time.

2. **Oats:** Oats are a great source of beta-glucan, a type of soluble fiber. This type of fiber can help reduce visceral fat by slowing down digestion and reducing the amount of fat absorbed by the body. It can also help to reduce blood sugar levels and improve insulin sensitivity. All of these factors can help to reduce visceral fat over time.

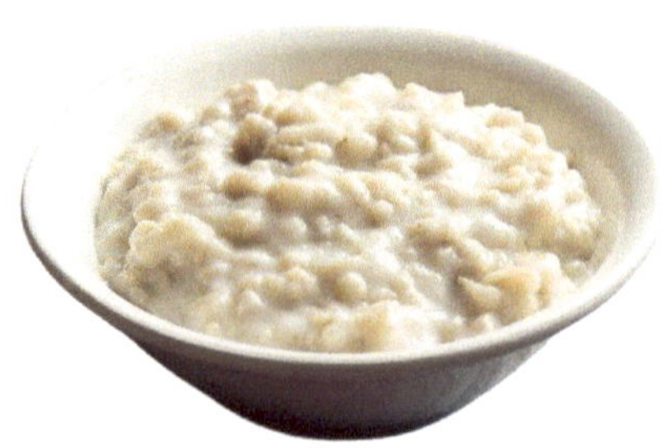

Oats are a versatile food that can be used in a variety of dishes. In addition to being a good source of beta-glucan, oats are also high in vitamins, minerals, and antioxidants. They're also a great source of complex carbohydrates, which provide long-lasting energy. And finally, they're low in calories and fat, making them a great choice for weight loss. some oat recipes are:

❖ **Overnight oats**: This is a simple, no-cook recipe that's perfect for busy mornings. All you need is some rolled oats, milk, yogurt, and your favorite toppings, like fruit, nuts, or seeds. Just mix all the ingredients together in a jar and let it sit overnight in the fridge. In the morning, you'll have a delicious and nutritious breakfast ready to go.

- ❖ **Baked oatmeal:** This is a hearty dish that's perfect for a weekend brunch. It's made with oats, milk, eggs, and your favorite add-ins, like berries, nuts, or chocolate chips. Just mix all the ingredients together and bake until golden brown. The result is a delicious and filling breakfast that's sure to keep you satisfied.

- ❖ **Savory oat pancakes:** These are a unique twist on traditional pancakes, and they're made with rolled oats, eggs, and other savory ingredients like cheese, scallions, and herbs. Just mix the ingredients together and cook like regular pancakes. They're perfect for a light dinner or as a side dish.

- ❖ **Oat crumble bars:** These bars are made with rolled oats, sugar, and butter, and they're filled with your favorite fruit, like apples, blueberries, or peaches. Just mix the ingredients together, press into a pan, and bake until golden brown. They're a delicious and healthier alternative to traditional dessert bars.

❖ **Oat energy bites:** These are perfect for a quick snack or an on-the-go breakfast. They're made with oats, nut butter, honey, and other ingredients like flaxseed, chia seeds, or dried fruit. Just mix the ingredients together, shape into balls, and store in the fridge. They're a great source of healthy fats, protein, and fiber.

3. **Greek yogurt:** Greek yogurt is an excellent source of protein, calcium, and probiotics, and it can be a great addition to a healthy diet. One way to enjoy Greek

yogurt is to add some fruit, nuts, and a drizzle of honey. This makes for a delicious and healthy snack or breakfast.

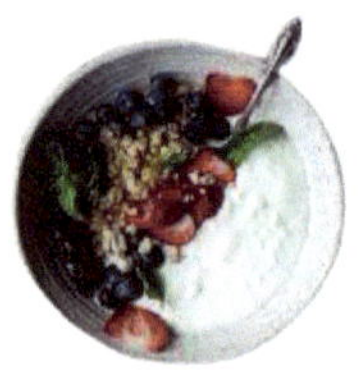 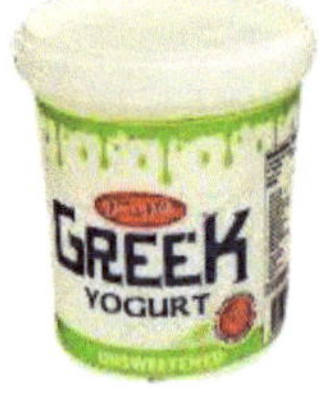 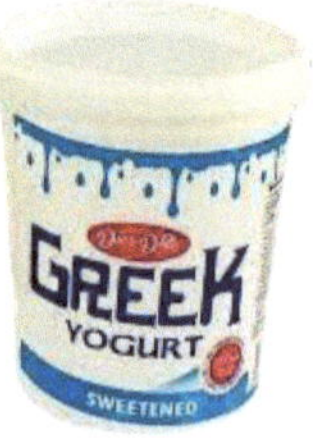

One of the best things about Greek yogurt is that it's a great source of protein. A single serving of Greek yogurt can have up to 20 grams of protein, which is more than many other types of yogurt. Protein is important for maintaining a healthy weight, muscle mass, and overall health. It's not just the protein that makes Greek yogurt a great choice. Greek yogurt is also a good source of calcium and probiotics. Calcium is important for bone health, and probiotics are beneficial for gut health. Greek yogurt is also low in lactose, making it a good choice for people who are lactose intolerant. So, it's not just the protein that makes Greek yogurt a healthy choice!

4. **Skinless chicken breast:** Skinless chicken breast is another great source of protein, and it's also a low-fat option. Chicken breast is leaner than other cuts of chicken, like thighs or drumsticks. A 3-ounce serving of skinless chicken breast has about 30 grams of protein and less than 3 grams of fat. That makes it a great choice for anyone looking to increase their protein intake without adding a lot of fat.

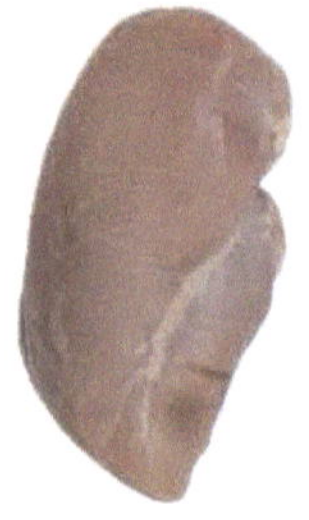 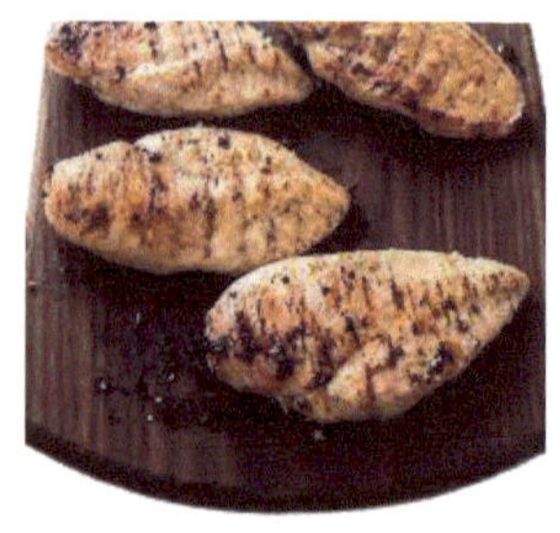

Eating foods that are high in protein, like chicken breast, can help reduce visceral fat in a few ways. First, protein helps to increase satiety, or the feeling of fullness. This can help to reduce overall calorie intake and promote weight loss. Second, protein helps to promote muscle growth and maintenance. Since muscle tissue burns more calories than fat tissue, this can also help to reduce visceral fat. Another benefit of eating chicken breast and other lean proteins, like fish and eggs. They can help to regulate blood sugar levels by slowing down the digestion and absorption of carbohydrates. This can help to keep blood sugar levels stable and reduce the risk of blood sugar spikes.

5. **Raspberries:** Raspberries are another great food for reducing visceral fat. They're not only delicious, but they're also a good source of fiber. A cup of raspberries has about 8 grams of fiber, which is about a third of the recommended daily intake for most adults. Fiber can help to promote weight loss by increasing satiety and slowing down digestion. Plus, raspberries are low in calories, so they're a great choice for anyone looking to lose weight or reduce visceral fat.

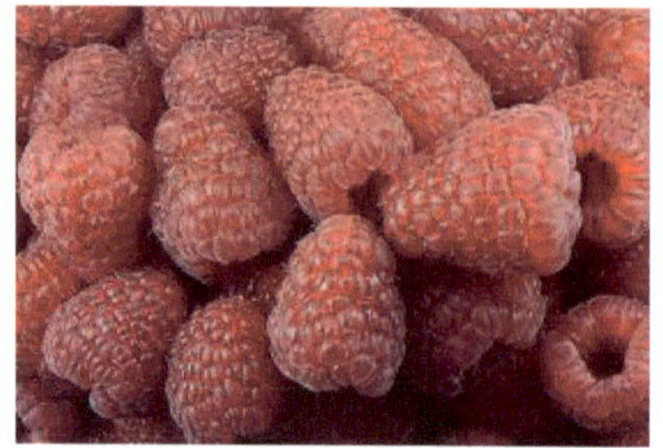

Raspberries are great source of antioxidants. These are compounds that can help to reduce inflammation and protect against disease. Some of the antioxidants found in raspberries include **anthocyanins, quercetin,** and **ellagic acid.** These antioxidants may help to reduce the risk of heart disease, cancer, and other chronic diseases. I'd like to add that raspberries are also a good source of vitamin C. Vitamin C is important for immune function, collagen production, and iron absorption. It's also a powerful antioxidant, so it can help to reduce inflammation and protect against disease.

6. **Lemons:** Lemons and other citrus fruits can help to reduce visceral fat in several ways. First, they can help to improve digestion, which can reduce bloating and gas. They can also help to control blood sugar levels, which can reduce cravings and promote weight loss. Finally, they can reduce inflammation, which is thought to play a role in the accumulation of visceral fat. So, adding lemons to your diet can be a great way to improve your overall health and reduce visceral fat.

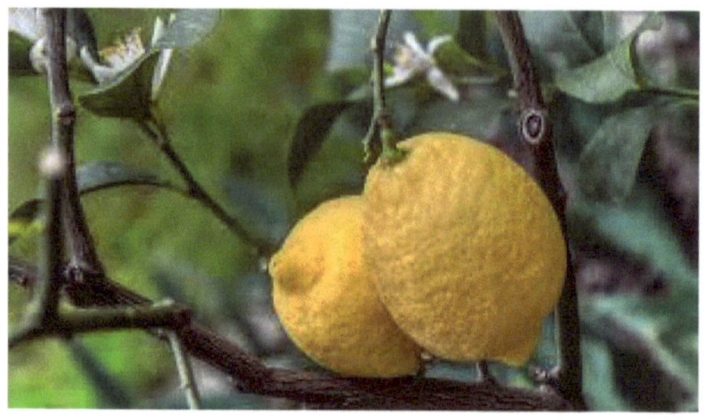

Lemons can also help to boost your metabolism. The citric acid in lemons can help to increase the breakdown of fat cells, and the vitamin C can help to boost the production of enzymes that are involved in fat burning. So, adding lemons to your diet can give your metabolism a little boost. One easy way to add lemons to your diet is to start your day with warm lemon water. Simply squeeze the juice of half a lemon into a glass of warm water and drink it first thing in the morning. This can help to kickstart your metabolism and get your digestion going. Another option is to add lemon juice to salad dressings, marinades, or smoothies. Another great way to get the benefits of lemons is to make a homemade lemon detox drink. This is made with lemon juice, warm water, and raw honey. Simply mix the ingredients together and drink it first thing in the morning. This can help to cleanse your system and give your metabolism a boost.

7. **Sprouted bread:** Sprouted bread is another great food for reducing visceral fat. This is because it's a whole grain bread that's easier to digest than traditional breads. This means that it's less likely

to cause bloating and gas. Additionally, sprouted bread is rich in fiber, which can help to reduce cravings and keep you feeling full.

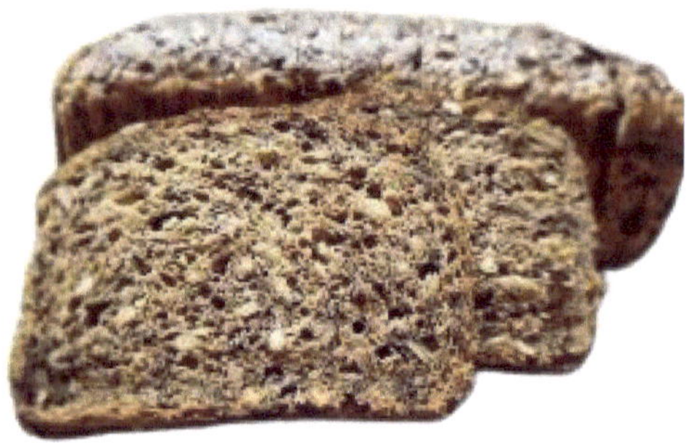

Sprouted bread is a versatile food that can be used in a variety of ways. You can use it to make sandwiches, toast, or even crackers. It's also a great option for those who are gluten-intolerant or have celiac disease.

**8. Avocados:** Avocados are great for reducing visceral fat. This is because they're high in monounsaturated fats, which are the "good" type of fat. Monounsaturated fats can help to increase feelings of fullness and reduce cravings. They can also improve cholesterol levels and reduce inflammation.

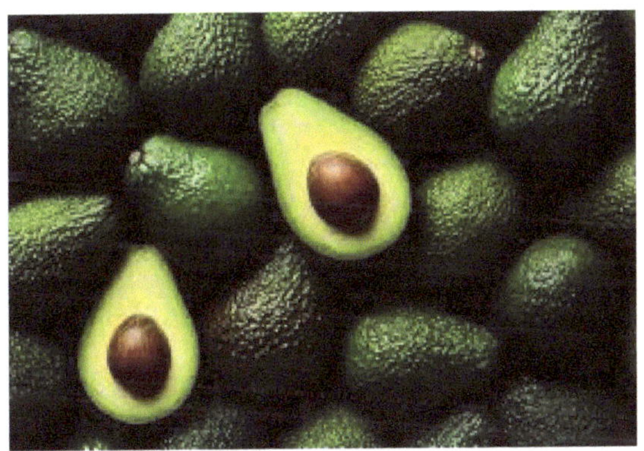

There are so many ways to enjoy avocados. You can add them to salads, sandwiches, or even smoothies. Or, you can make homemade guacamole with avocados, lime juice, cilantro, and a bit of salt. You can even use avocados as a healthy substitute for butter or oil in baking recipes.

9. **Eggs:** Another great food for reducing visceral fat are eggs. This is because they're a good source of protein and healthy fats. They're also high in choline, which is a nutrient that's important for fat metabolism. And, studies have shown that people who eat eggs for breakfast tend to eat fewer calories throughout the day.

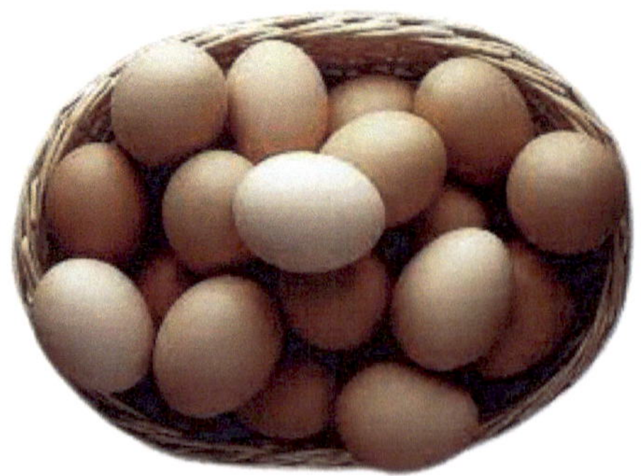

Since a lot of people seem to be liking the idea of eggs for breakfast, I'll share a recipe with you. How about egg muffins? These are made with eggs, veggies, and a bit of cheese. They're easy to make and can be eaten on the go. Simply mix the ingredients together and bake them in a muffin tin. Then, you can store them in the fridge and eat them throughout the week.

10. **Salmon:** This is another excellent food for reducing visceral fat. It's a great source of protein and omega-3 fatty acids, which are beneficial for heart health and weight loss. Omega-3 fatty acids may also help to reduce inflammation and improve insulin sensitivity.

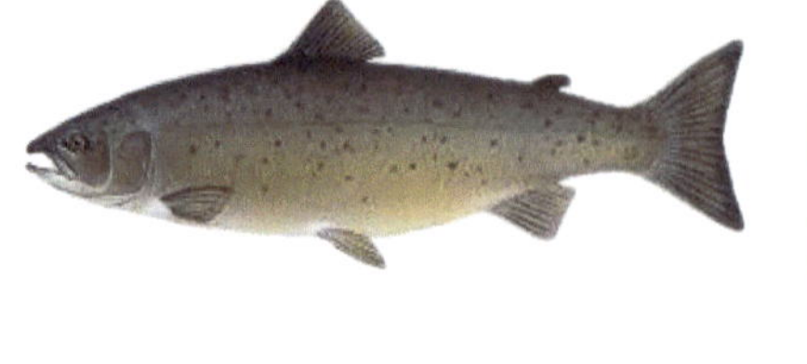 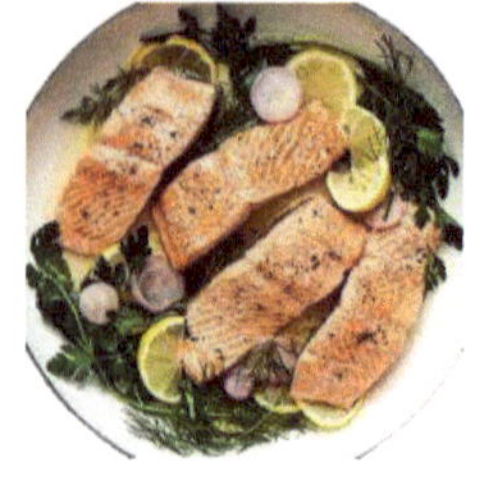

There are many ways to enjoy salmon. You can bake, broil, or grill it. You can also make salmon burgers, which are a delicious and healthy alternative to traditional hamburgers. And, you can add canned salmon to salads, pasta dishes, and casseroles. Another recipe with you for salmon with lemon and dill. This is a simple recipe that only takes about 20 minutes to make. Simply season the salmon with salt and pepper, and then cook it in a skillet. Once it's cooked, squeeze some lemon juice over it and sprinkle it with fresh dill.

11.**Quinoa:** Quinoa is a grain-like seed that's become increasingly popular in recent years. It's a good source of protein and fiber, and it's also gluten-free. Additionally, quinoa is high in magnesium, which may help to reduce visceral fat. And, it's a versatile ingredient that can be used in a variety of dishes.

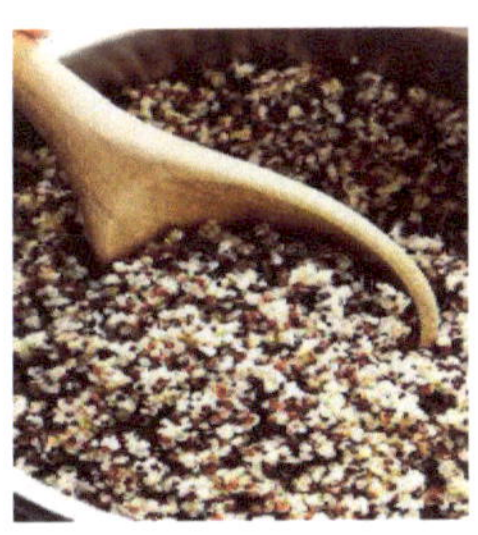 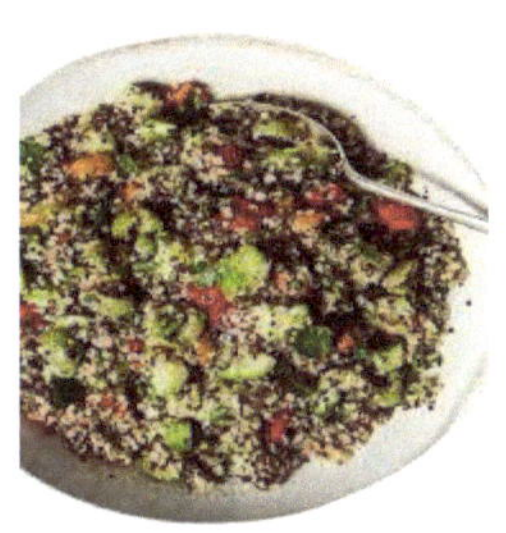

A good example of quinoa recipe is, quinoa and black bean burgers; These are made with quinoa, black beans, egg, garlic, and spices. They're easy to make and packed with protein and fiber. Plus, they're a great option for vegetarians and vegans.

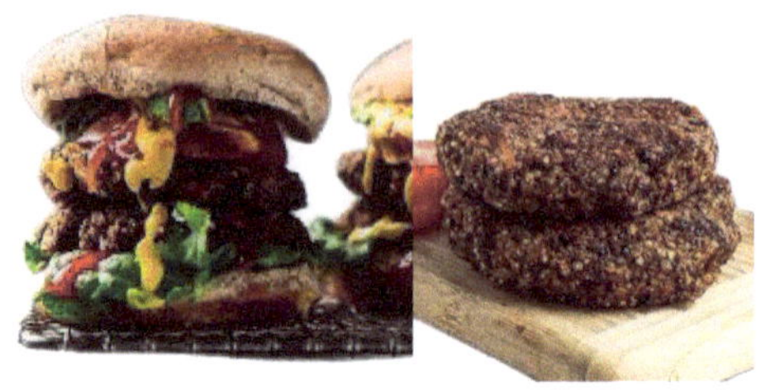

**12.Green tea:** Green tea is a great choice for reducing visceral fat because it contains a compound called catechins. Catechins are antioxidants that may boost metabolism and increase fat burning. A good example of green tea is matcha. Matcha is a powdered form of green tea that contains higher levels of catechins than regular green tea. Matcha can be made into a latte or added to smoothies.

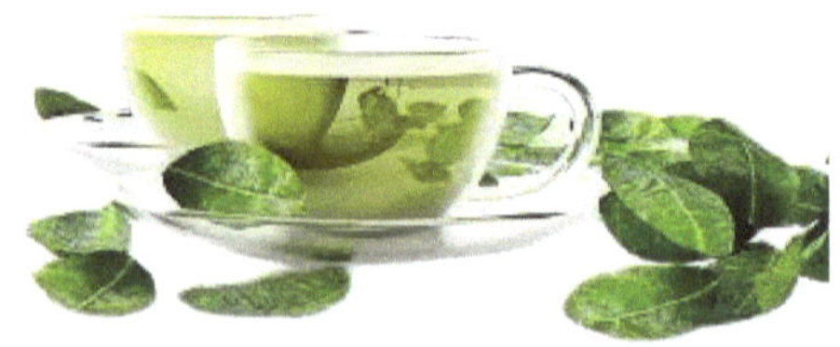

13. **Water with lemon:** Lemon water is a simple and refreshing way to boost your hydration and help reduce visceral fat. Lemon water also has vitamin C and antioxidants. Drinking water with lemon is that it can help with digestion. The acidity in the lemon helps to stimulate the production of digestive enzymes, which can improve digestion and reduce bloating. Lemon water can also help to alkalize the body, which can help reduce visceral fat.

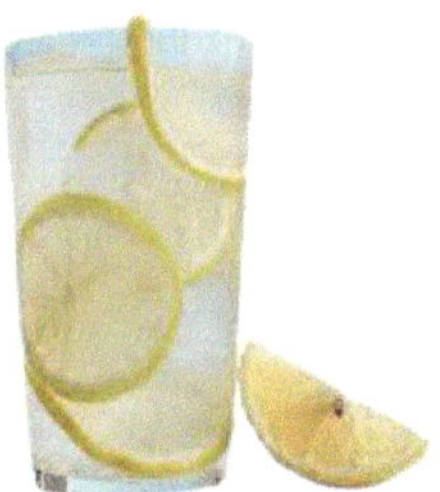

14. **Cottage cheese:** Cottage cheese is a <u>curdled</u> milk product with a mild flavour and a creamy,

heterogeneous, soupy texture, made from <u>skimmed milk</u>. An essential step in the manufacturing process distinguishing cottage cheese from other fresh cheeses is the addition of a "dressing" to the curd grains, usually <u>cream</u>, which is mainly responsible for the taste of the product.

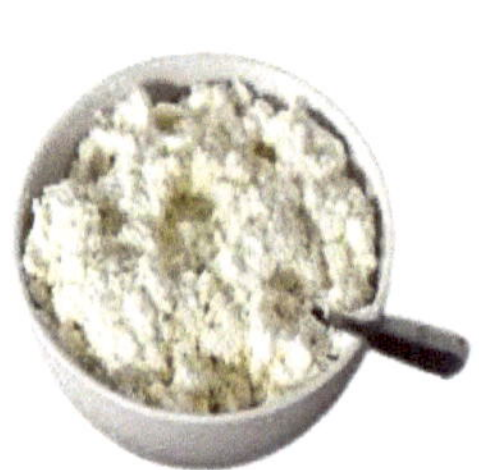
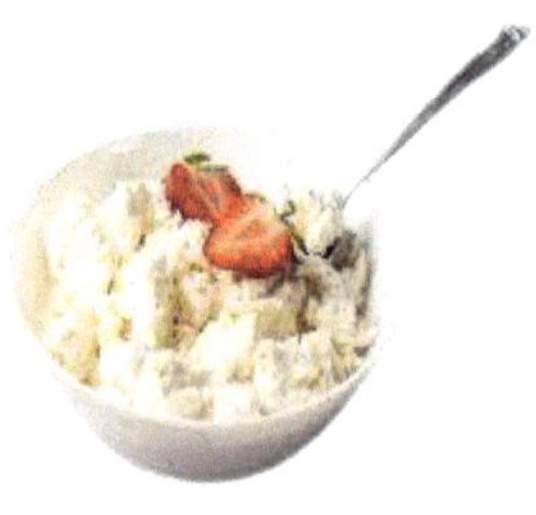

Cottage cheese can be low in <u>calories</u> compared to other types of cheese — similar to <u>yogurt</u>; this makes it popular among dieters and some health devotees. It can be used with various foods such as yogurt, fruit, toast, and granola, in salads, as a dip, and as a replacement for mayonnaise. Cottage cheese is a good source of protein and calcium, and it's low in calories. One serving of cottage cheese provides about 14 grams of protein, making it a great option for a quick and healthy snack. It also contains probiotics, which can help to improve gut health. You can add some berries and a drizzle of honey for a sweet and satisfying snack. Or, you could add some chopped herbs and a squeeze of lemon for a savory option. Cottage cheese can also be used as a topping for toast or as a base for a veggie dip.

**15. Black Beans:** Black beans are another nutritious food that can help reduce visceral fat. They're a great source of protein, fiber, and other nutrients like magnesium and iron. Black beans can be added to salads, soups, or even baked goods. They can also be mashed and used as a dip for veggies or chips. One of the best things about black beans is that they're a great source of resistant starch. Resistant starch is a type of carbohydrate that's not easily digested and absorbed by the body. Instead, it ends up in the large intestine, where it acts like a prebiotic and feeds the good bacteria in the gut.

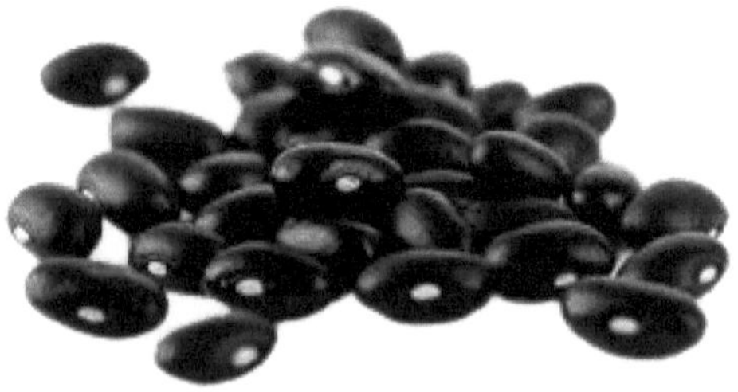

This can help to improve gut health and reduce visceral fat. Another thing to know about black beans is that they can help regulate blood sugar levels. The fiber and resistant starch in black beans can slow down the digestion and absorption of carbohydrates, which can prevent blood sugar spikes. This can help to improve insulin sensitivity and reduce the risk of type 2 diabetes. Black beans are a versatile and nutritious ingredient that can be used in a variety of recipes. One delicious way to enjoy black beans is in a black bean and sweet potato chili. This hearty chili is made with black beans, sweet potatoes, onions, bell peppers, tomatoes, and a blend of spices. It's healthy, filling, and packed with fl

**16. Tuna:** Tuna is another food that's great for reducing visceral fat. It's high in protein and omega-3 fatty acids, which can help to increase satiety and reduce inflammation. Tuna can be enjoyed in a variety of ways, including as a sandwich filling, as a topping for salads, or even as sushi. Tuna is a lean protein that's low in calories and fat, which makes it a great choice for weight loss. It's also rich in B vitamins, which are important for energy production and metabolism. And, it's a good source of selenium, which is important for immune function and thyroid health. Tuna is also versatile and easy to prepare.

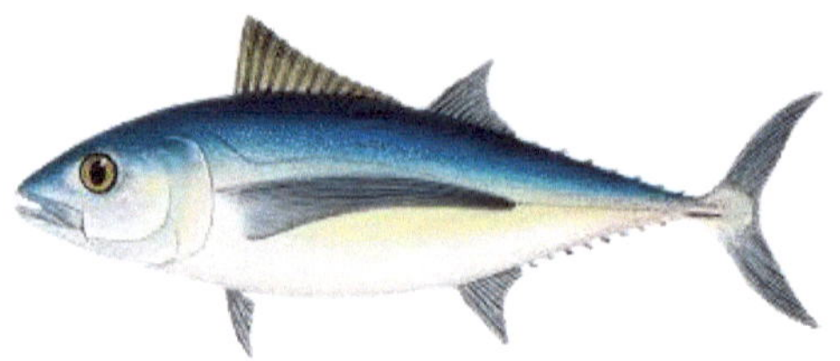

Another reason to love tuna: it's a fast-digesting protein. This means that it's absorbed quickly by the body, which can help to promote muscle growth and recovery after exercise. So, if you're looking for a quick and easy post-workout snack, tuna is a great choice.

**17. Jicama:** Jicama! It's a root vegetable that's native to Mexico. It's a good source of fiber, vitamin C, and potassium. It has a sweet and crunchy texture, making it a great option for salads, slaws, and even as a chip replacement. And, because of its high fiber content, it can help to promote weight loss and reduce visceral fat. Jicama is a versatile vegetable that can be enjoyed raw or cooked. Raw jicama can be sliced and added to salads or enjoyed as a snack

with a bit of lime juice and chili powder. It can also
be cooked and added to soups, stews, or stir-fries.
Another fun way to enjoy jicama is to slice it thin
and use it as a wrap for fillings like chicken or
shrimp. Jicama can be a great way to add variety and
nutrition to your meals.

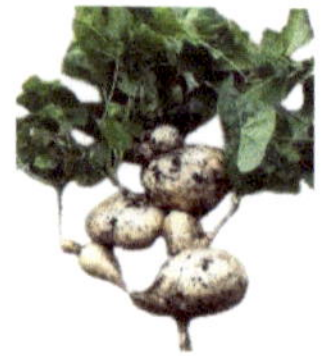 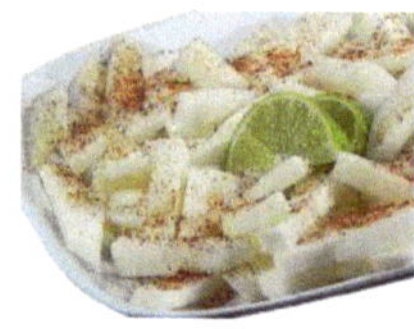 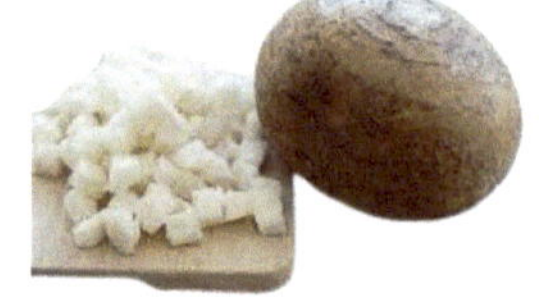

Jicama is a low-calorie food that's also low in
sugar, making it a great choice for people with
diabetes or who are watching their blood sugar
levels. It's also versatile and easy to prepare. One
fun way to enjoy jicama is to use it as the base for
a "taco shell." Simply slice the jicama thin and fill
it with taco fillings like ground beef, shredded

lettuce, and salsa. This is a healthier and more nutritious alternative to traditional taco shells.

18. **Edamame:** Edamame is another great food for reducing visceral fat. It's a soybean that's harvested when it's still green and immature. Edamame is a good source of protein, fiber, and other nutrients like iron and magnesium. It's often served as an appetizer at Japanese restaurants, but it can also be added to salads, stir-fries, or even eaten as a snack. Like jicama, edamame is low in calories and high in fiber, making it a great choice for weight loss and healthy eating. One of the best things about edamame is that it's a complete protein, meaning that it contains all nine essential amino acids. This makes it a great option for

vegans and vegetarians, as well as anyone looking to increase their protein intake. Edamame is also low in fat and cholesterol-free, making it a healthy snack option. You can enjoy edamame either fresh or frozen. To prepare fresh edamame, simply boil it for a few minutes and then sprinkle it with sea salt.

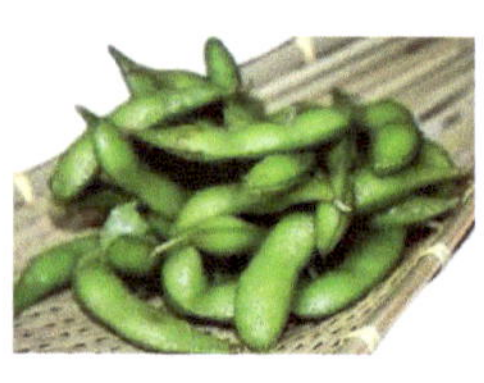 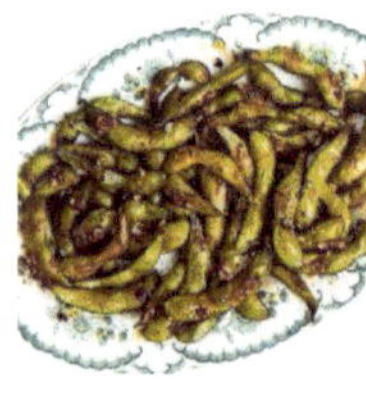 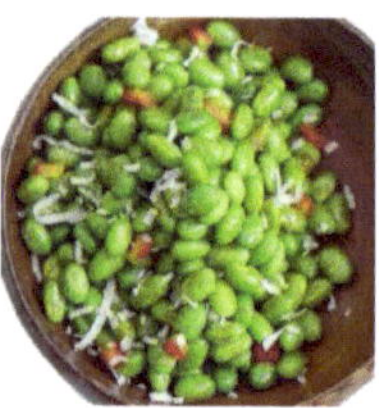

Another interesting fact about edamame is that it contains isoflavones, which are phytoestrogens found in plants. These compounds have been shown to have a protective effect against chronic diseases like heart disease, cancer, and osteoporosis. So, not only is edamame a healthy and delicious snack, but it may also have some health benefits that go beyond weight loss and fat reduction.

## specific meal ideas that can help reduce visceral fat.

- For breakfast, consider eating oatmeal with berries, yogurt, and a small handful of nuts. For lunch, try a salad with chicken, quinoa, and plenty of veggies. And for dinner, try a bowl of brown rice, grilled salmon, and a big side of veggies.

- Now let's talk about another key component of a healthy diet: healthy fats. Healthy fats, like omega-3 fatty acids, can actually help reduce visceral fat. Omega-3 fatty acids are found in foods like salmon, walnuts, flaxseeds, and chia seeds. These fats are also anti-inflammatory, which means they can help reduce the risk of heart disease and other chronic diseases. Are you getting enough healthy fats in your diet?

- Another key recipes of a healthy diet: fiber. Fiber is important for digestive health, and it can also help reduce visceral fat. Fiber is found in many plant-based foods, like whole grains, fruits, and vegetables. Aim to get 25-30 grams of fiber per day.

- You can also aim for at least five servings of fruits and vegetables per day. Fruits and vegetables are packed with vitamins, minerals, and antioxidants, all of which are important for your health. They're also a great source of fiber. Let me break it down for you. Let's say you have a banana with breakfast, an apple for a snack, and a salad with dinner. That's already three servings of fruits and veggies! The remaining two servings could come from a side of broccoli with lunch, and a small bowl of berries for dessert. Hope that help to visualize how you could reach the goal of five servings per day?

- Now, let's talk about another important dietary factor: hydration. Staying well-hydrated is essential for your overall health, and it can also help reduce visceral fat. Aim to drink at least eight glasses of water per day.

**Intermittent fasting:**

One more dietary factor I'd like to discuss:

intermittent fasting. This is when you eat within a certain time frame each day, and fast for the rest of the day. For example, you might eat only between 8 AM and 6 PM, and then fast for the rest of the day. Intermittent fasting can take a few different forms. One common approach is called the 16:8 method, which means fasting for 16 hours and eating within an 8-hour window. For example, you might eat between 12 PM and 8 PM, and fast for the remaining 16 hours. This can be a bit challenging at first, but it can become easier with time. Another common type of intermittent fasting is called the 5:2 method. This involves eating normally five days a week and then eating very little (only about 500-600 calories) on the remaining two days. For example, you might eat normally on Monday through Friday and then fast on Saturday and Sunday. Let's also mention the one-meal-a-day (OMAD) method, which is pretty much what it sounds like - eating all of your food within a one-hour window each day. It's a more extreme form of intermittent fasting, but some people find it effective. Some research suggests that intermittent fasting may help reduce visceral fat.

# CHAPTER THREE

## Simple exercise to do at home to reduce visceral fat

Now that you've learned about some of the foods that can help to reduce visceral fat, it's time to talk about exercise. Exercise is an important part of any weight loss or fat reduction program, and there are plenty of simple exercises that you can do at home to help reduce visceral fat. Read on to learn more about these exercises and how they can help you achieve your goals.

1. **SQUATS:** Squats are a great exercise for reducing visceral fat because they work the large muscle groups in the lower body, which helps to boost the metabolism and burn more calories. You can start with bodyweight squats and then progress to weighted squats once you've

mastered the form. Sure thing! Squats are an excellent exercise for the lower body and core, and they can help to improve strength, balance, and flexibility. When performing a squat, it's important to maintain proper form to avoid injury. Here are some tips for doing a bodyweight squat:

➢ Stand with your feet shoulder-width apart, with your arms extended straight in front of you for balance.

➢ Slowly bend your knees and lower your hips, as if you're sitting down in a chair.

➢ Keep your chest up, your back straight, and your core engaged.

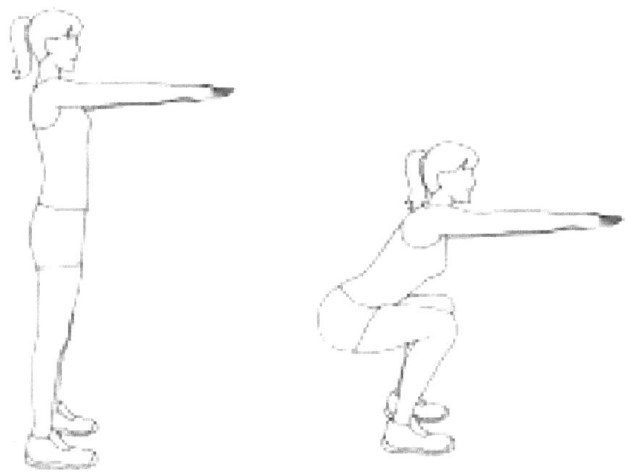

To progress to weighted squats, you can use dumbbells, kettlebells, or a barbell. Start with a light weight and gradually increase the weight as you get stronger. Here are some tips for performing a weighted squat:

➤ Start by standing with your feet shoulder-width apart, with the weight resting on your shoulders or across your upper back.

➢ Squat down, keeping your chest up and your weight back in your heels.

➢ Pause at the bottom of the squat, then push through your heels to stand back up.

2. **Push-ups:** another exercise that's great for reducing visceral fat: push-ups. Push-ups are a compound exercise that work multiple muscle groups, including the chest, shoulders, triceps, and core. They can be done with or without weight, and there are several variations that can make them more challenging. Push-ups are a classic bodyweight exercise that can be done almost anywhere, making them a great option for at-home workouts. To perform a standard push-

up, start in a high plank position with your hands shoulder-width apart and your body in a straight line from head to heels. Lower your chest towards the ground, then push back up to the starting position. It's important to keep your core engaged and your body in a straight line throughout the movement.

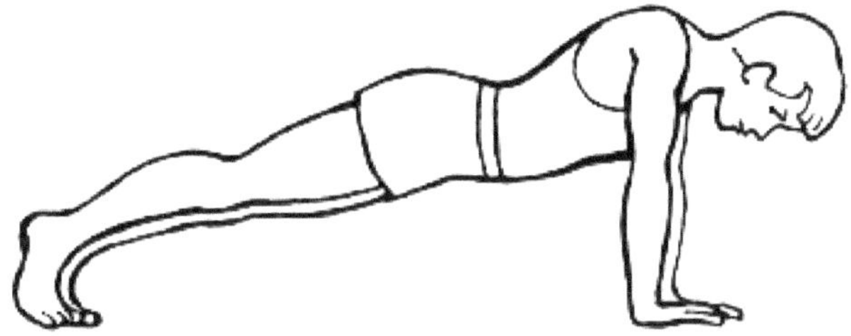

Variations of the push-up that can help to target different muscle groups. For example, you can try a wide grip push-up, which targets the outer chest muscles. Or, you can try a close grip push-up, which targets the triceps. You can also add weight to your push-ups by wearing a weighted vest or using resistance bands.

3. **THE PLANK:** The plank is a core exercise that can help to strengthen the abdominal muscles and improve posture. It can be done on your elbows or your hands, and there are several variations that can make it more challenging. For example, you can try a side plank or a weighted plank.

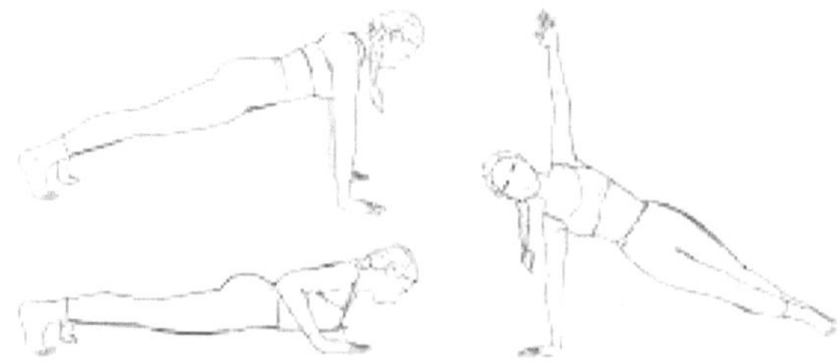

The plank is a simple exercise that can be done anywhere, making it a great option for at-home workouts. To perform a standard plank, start in a high plank position with your hands shoulder-width apart and your body in a straight line from head to heels. Hold this position for as long as you can, keeping your core engaged and your hips level with the ground. Aim to hold the plank for 30 seconds to start, and gradually increase the duration as you get stronger.

4. **THE BURPEE:** The burpee is a full-body exercise that combines a squat, a plank, and a jump. It's a challenging exercise that can help to improve your cardiovascular fitness and burn calories. Here's how to do a burpee:

- Start in a standing position and quickly squat down, placing your hands on the ground in front of you.

- Kick your legs back into a high plank position.

- Quickly return to a squat position, then jump up as high as you can.

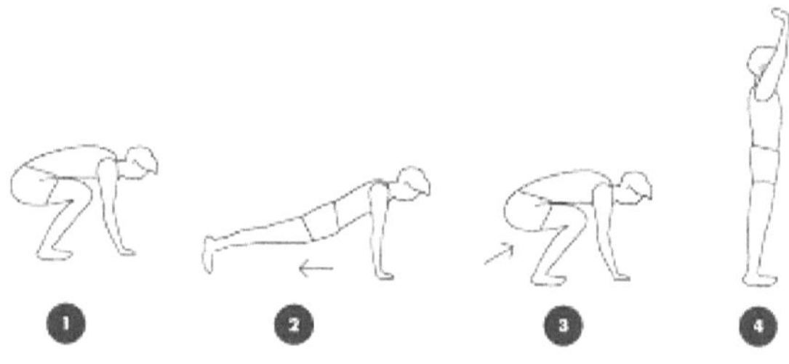

## Tips for doing a burpee with proper form:

- Make sure to keep your back straight and your core engaged throughout the movement.

- Be sure to land with soft knees when you jump.

- Focus on your breath. Exhale as you jump, and inhale as you squat down.

- If the full burpee is too challenging, you can modify the exercise by stepping your feet back one at a time, rather than jumping back into a high plank position.

5. **MOUNTAIN CLIMBERS:** Mountain climbers are a cardio and core exercise that can help to improve your endurance and burn calories. To do mountain climbers, start in a high plank position with your hands shoulder-width apart and your body in a straight line from head to

heels. Bring one knee towards your chest, then quickly switch and bring the other knee towards your chest. Keep your core engaged and your hips level with the ground throughout the movement.

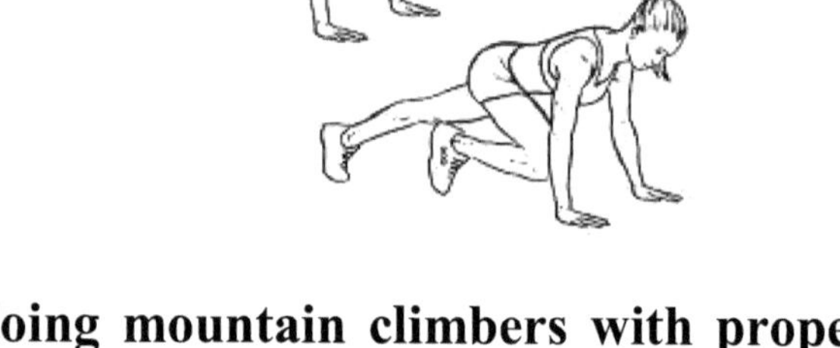

## Tips for doing mountain climbers with proper form:

- Focus on keeping your hips low and your core tight.

- If you're having trouble keeping your balance, try slowing down the movement or keeping your knees closer to the ground.

- To increase the intensity, you can try bringing your knees to your chest faster or even adding a hop in between each rep.

- To make the exercise easier, you can start with one knee at a time.

❖ Now that we've covered some exercises that can help to reduce visceral fat, let's talk about **how to incorporate these exercises into your workout routine.** For maximum results, try doing these exercises at least three times per week. You can also add in other exercises like jogging or cycling for additional cardio. It's never too late to start a fitness routine. The key is to start slow and gradually increase the intensity over time. If you're just starting out, try doing each exercise for 30 seconds and then resting for 30 seconds. Gradually increase the duration of each exercise and reduce the rest time over time. And remember, consistency is key! Try to make exercise a part of your daily routine, even if it's just for a few minutes each day.

# CHAPTER FOUR

## Stress management techniques and how they relate to visceral fat

As we've discussed, there are several factors that can contribute to the accumulation of visceral fat, including diet, exercise, and sleep. However, another important factor that can impact visceral fat is stress. When you're stressed, your body releases the stress hormone cortisol, which can cause fat to accumulate around the midsection. Therefore, managing stress is an important part of reducing visceral fat. Below are some stress management techniques that can help reduce visceral fat:

a. **Meditation:** Meditation is an ancient practice that has been shown to have numerous benefits for physical and mental health. By focusing your attention and clearing your mind, meditation can help you to reduce stress and anxiety. In addition, research has shown that regular meditation can help to lower cortisol levels, which can reduce the accumulation of visceral fat. Practicing meditation can help reduce stress levels and improve overall mental health.

b. **Deep Breathing:** Deep breathing is a simple yet powerful technique that can help to reduce stress and promote relaxation. When you take slow, deep breaths, you activate the parasympathetic nervous system, which helps to slow down your heart rate and lower your blood pressure. This can help to calm the mind and relax the body, reducing stress and helping to prevent the accumulation of visceral fat. You can practice deep breathing at any time, even when you're feeling stressed or anxious.

c. **Exercise:** Exercise is not only a great way to stay physically fit, but it can also be a powerful stress-reliever. When you exercise, your body releases endorphins, which are feel-good chemicals that can improve your mood and reduce stress. In addition, exercise can help to improve sleep quality and reduce cortisol levels, which can help to reduce visceral fat. If you're feeling stressed, try going for a walk, doing some yoga, or hitting the gym for a workout.

d. **Time management:** Organizing your time can help you feel more in control and less stressed. Poor time management can lead to stress and anxiety, as you may feel overwhelmed by all the tasks on your plate. By organizing your time and setting priorities, you can reduce stress and feel more in control of your life. Try using a planner or scheduling app to keep track of your commitments and deadlines. You can also try setting aside a specific time each day for relaxation, such as reading a book or taking a bath. By taking control of your time, you can reduce stress and prevent the accumulation of visceral fat.

**Note:** *Stress management is a vital component of reducing visceral fat. By incorporating meditation, deep breathing, exercise, and time management into your daily routine, you can reduce stress and prevent the accumulation of visceral fat. By taking* *care of your mental health, you can improve your physical health and reduce the risk of chronic diseases like heart disease and diabetes. Remember, your mind and body are deeply connected, and taking care of both will help you achieve a healthier and happier life.*

# CHAPTER FIVE

## Summary and call to action

The accumulation of visceral fat is a serious health concern that can lead to a number of chronic diseases. However, by following the guidelines and techniques outlined in this book, you can take control of your health and reduce visceral fat. From adopting healthy eating habits and exploring new recipes to incorporating simple at-home exercises and stress management techniques into your daily routine, you have a range of options for reducing your visceral fat and improving your overall well-being.

## NOTE:

Remember, reducing visceral fat is not a one-time event.

❖ Now that you've learned about the steps you can take to reduce visceral fat and improve your health, it's time to commit to making positive changes in your life. Start by setting realistic goals and making small, sustainable changes to your diet and exercise routine. For example, you might commit to eating more vegetables and fruits, or you might decide to take a daily walk.

❖ The most important thing is to be patient with yourself and remember that progress takes time. Be kind to yourself and celebrate your successes along the way. You have the power to improve your health and reduce visceral fat, and you deserve to feel your best.

You now have the knowledge and tools to take charge of your health and reduce visceral fat. Remember, every small step you take towards improving your health is a victory worth celebrating. So, make a commitment to yourself today and start

# ABOUT THE AUTHOR

Dr. Devon M. C. is a health and wellness enthusiast with a passion for helping people live their best lives. He has a deep understanding of the factors that contribute to visceral fat accumulation and how to reduce it through simple lifestyle changes. His writing is engaging, approachable, and packed with practical advice that anyone can follow. When he's not writing, Dr. Devon enjoys staying active and trying new recipes that are both delicious and nutritious.